Eating Clean For Weight Loss

Natural Weight Management from Eating Healthy Whole Foods

RON KNESS

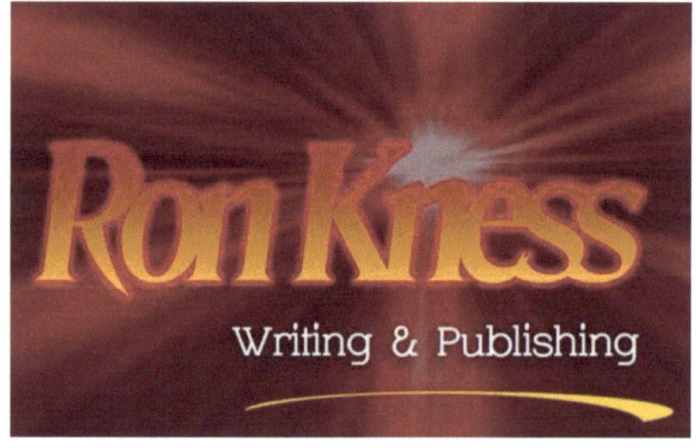

https://ronknesswriting.com

Contents

Disclaimer

This publication is for informational purposes only and is not intended as medical advice. Medical advice should always be obtained from a qualified medical professional for any health conditions or symptoms associated with them.

Every possible effort has been made in preparing and researching this material. We make no warranties with respect to the accuracy, applicability of its contents or any omissions.

See your healthcare professional before starting any diet, health or exercise program!

Introduction

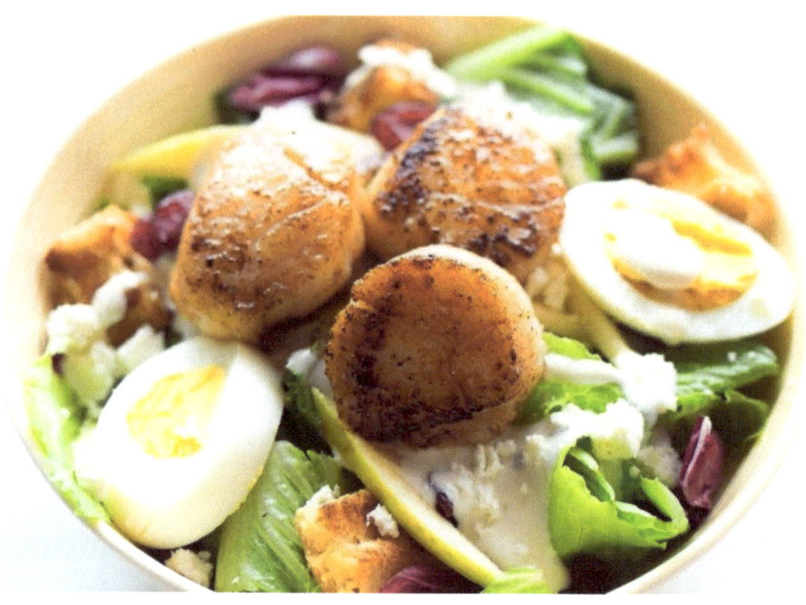

It is more and more difficult today to know everything you are putting into your body when you eat food. Between chemicals added to preserve freshness, hormones injected to promote growth, antibiotics given to stave off infection, and unhealthy fats added to enhance shelf life, today's foods are often more science than nature. That's where clean eating helps.

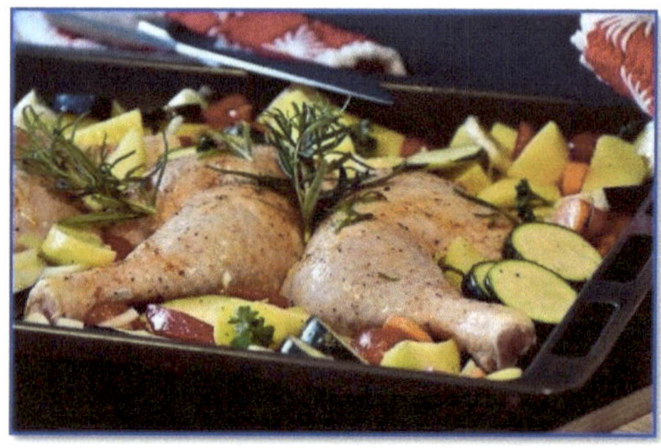

Keep reading to learn all about what clean eating is, why it is important for you and your health, how clean eating can help you lose weight and maintain your loss, and what foods are included in a clean eating plan.

We'll even help you make the transition to clean eating with some helpful tips that will keep you on the right track. Our complete guide to clean eating tells you everything you ever wanted to know about this approach to food.

Just What Is Clean Eating?

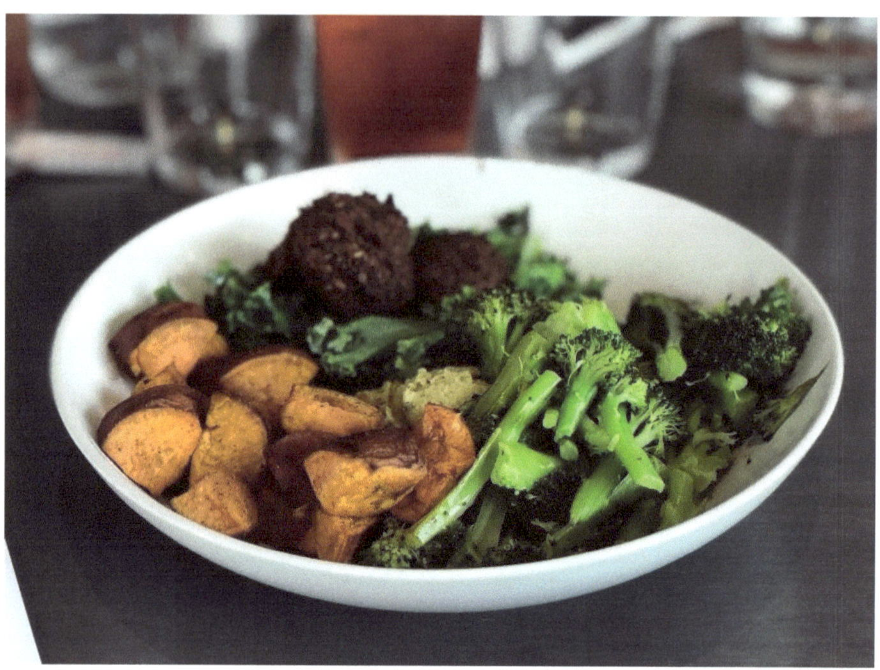

There is no need to make any explanation of clean eating complicated. Clean eating is about mindfully selecting foods that are whole or minimally refined or processed, leaving them closer to their natural form. This way of eating is in contrast to other "diets" that promote counting carbs or fat or protein and instead allows you to eat a variety of foods that are just that- food.

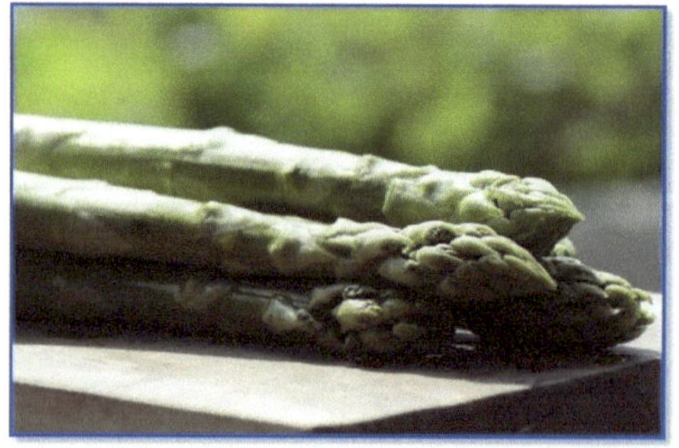

No chemicals, no preservatives, very few alterations from its original form.

Unfortunately, our society's approach to eating, and the food production that supplies our food makes it challenging to eat clean.

If you want to make a move to eating clean, the first thing you have to understand is that, yes, it is about your diet and how you eat, but it isn't necessarily a "diet" as we come to think of that word today.

Instead, clean eating is about making lifestyle choices that will enhance your health. You aren't going to drop 50 pounds in one month when you eat clean. Instead, you will be making more nutritious choices about what you put in your body, and you will be more mindful of the foods you eat.

Because eating clean is about reducing processed foods, that means you will naturally eat fewer carbohydrates, unhealthy fats, and sugars. This, in turn, will have many positive effects on your body, including weight loss if you are overweight.

Eating clean means, you value your body and your health so much that you select only the very best fuel to power you throughout each day.

A clean eating approach means you are removing the junk food that has come to be a large part of the Western diet, sometimes called the Standard American Diet, or SAD. It is *sad* indeed. Instead of eating foods with artificial flavors, refined sugars, excess amounts of salt, you eat whole foods that are not processed, refined, packaged, or *enhanced* with artificial ingredients.

What you *do* enjoy with a clean-eating approach is tons of fresh vegetables and fruits, healthy fats, lean proteins, and unrefined grains.

With a focus on the quality of your food, you won't have to obsess over the quantity in order to lose weight and be healthy. Combined with an active lifestyle, a clean eating approach to food will have numerous health benefits, will leave you feeling satisfied, and will keep you in touch with where your food comes from.

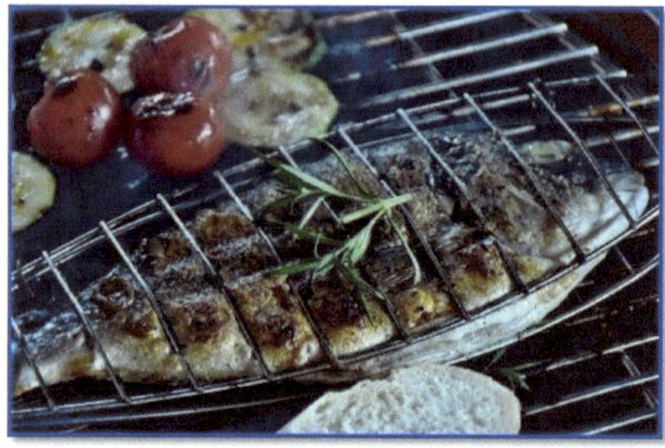

There is not one set approach to clean eating. Some tout strict adherence to specific rules, while others follow different guidelines. Finding what is realistic and healthy for you will be necessary to make this approach to eating work for you and to make it a lasting part of your lifestyle.

Without that, you will end up feeling deprived or unhappy and revert to former, less healthy ways of eating. We offer hints and strategies for making clean eating work for you, but you must decide on the best approach to this lifestyle for your own health and needs.

Many will find that the clean eating approach is preferable to other ways of eating because it is not a traditional diet. It does not involve counting anything, restricting how much you eat, or depriving yourself of tastes you love. It's just about being more in tune with your food choices, using less processed and artificial ingredients, and learning to love food for its health benefits.

If you are looking to lose weight through a clean eating approach, you are in luck. Keep reading to learn more about how clean eating can help you shed pounds and improve your weight loss efforts.

Let's Talk About Processed Foods

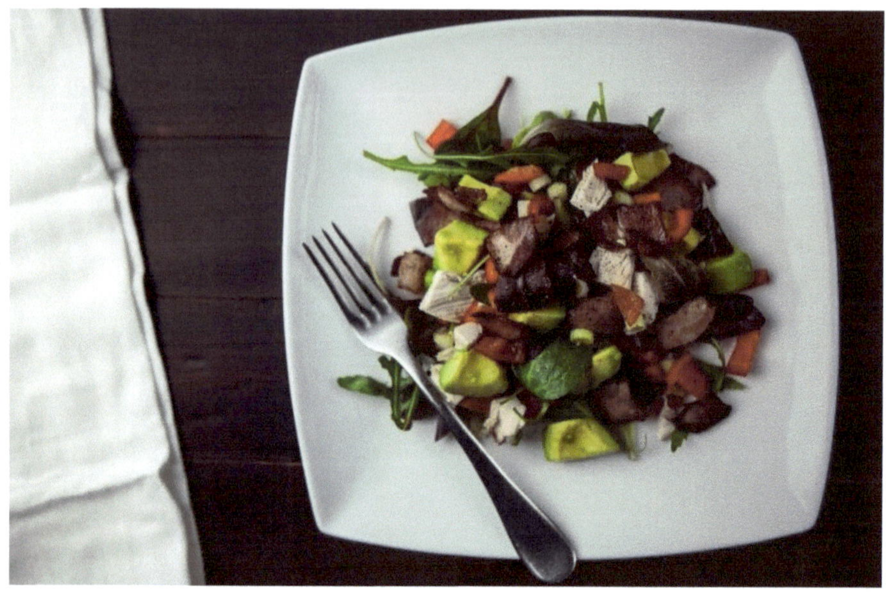

First, let's consider what we really mean when we talk about processed foods. Processing foods can have a number of different effects on the food itself, which in turn affects our bodies in significant ways. So, what is processed food?

This includes any of the following:

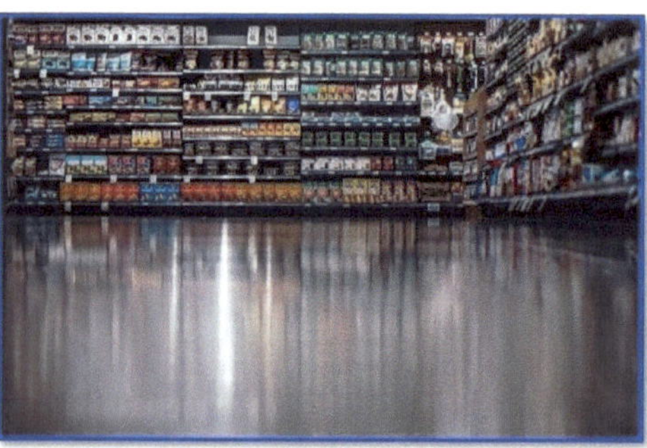

- Anything added to food to enhance flavor, improve shelf life, change the mouthfeel, make the food last longer, add extra vitamins, or change the color of a food.

This includes added sugar, fat, and salt, as well as all sorts of ingredients with often unrecognizable names.

- Refinements that change the form of the food, including removing part of grains such as the germ

- Any ingredient or component that is manufactured rather than grown

What About Cooking?

In reality, any form of cooking is also processing, so everything from making apples into applesauce to sautéing vegetables could be considered processing foods. However, eating a raw-food diet isn't for everyone nor is it necessary to stick with a clean eating approach. It's all about a spectrum or processing.

Here's an example.

Let's say you want a marinara sauce for your dinner tonight.

One option would be to purchase a jar of sauce from the store. As long as that jar contains more than a few ingredients, it is likely not a clean choice.

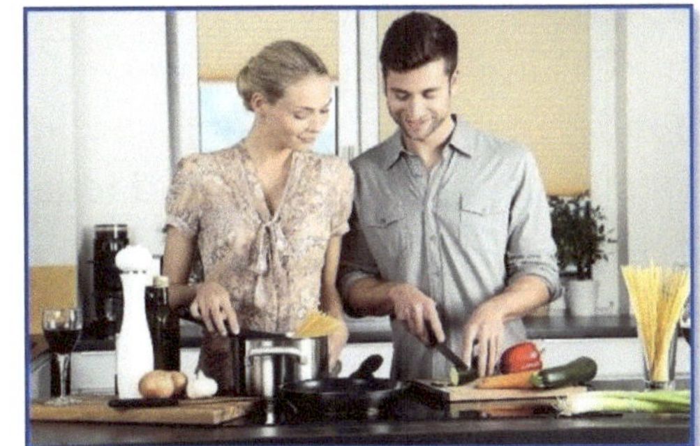

The second option is to purchase a jar that contains organic tomatoes, a few herbs and spices, and that's it. No added sugars, salt, or other ingredients.

This is a cleaner yet choice. The third and cleanest option is to purchase fresh tomatoes, basil, garlic, and herbs to make your own sauce. This option is the cleanest, but it is still processed, because you are cooking the foods and changing them from their original form.

The ideas behind clean eating are to process foods as minimally as possible and still make them enjoyable and healthy. Not all processing of foods is inherently bad. In fact, cooking certain foods releases nutrients we would not normally have access to in their raw form.

Cooking removes bacteria and toxins. Cooking gives us access to foods when they are out of season through freezing and canning. Cooking changes the consistency of foods, making them easier to digest and more appealing to our palates.

These types of processing actions are not categorically bad, so stop worrying that clean eating means only raw food.

The above examples of processed foods are ones you can include, in moderation, in a clean eating approach, along with other, less-processed foods. What you want to avoid entirely, are the highly-processed, or ultra-processed, foods found so commonly in kitchens, grocery stores, and restaurants around the world today.

The Miracle of Whole Foods

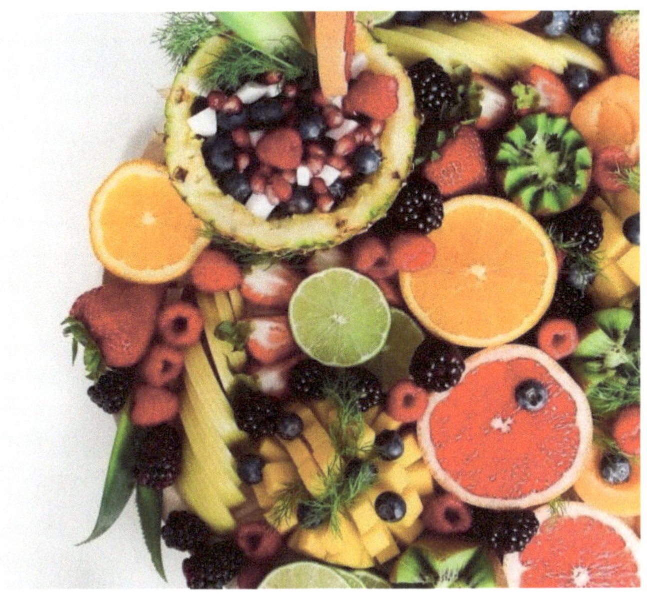

Whole food is the star of clean eating and is food that is eaten in its natural state without any processing.

According to Tara Gidus, RD, whole foods are foods "in [their] natural state" that are "intact, with all of the vitamins, minerals, and other nutrients that are in the food."

WebMD makes the distinction of whole food clear, an apple versus apple pie, a plain baked potato versus potato chips, or a grilled chicken breast versus chicken nugget. Additionally, whole foods don't have to be organic or pesticide-free, though in some cases these are good choices.

Energy Dense Versus Nutrient Dense

There are two types of foods, nutrient dense foods and energy dense foods, and that is the quintessential difference between whole and processed foods.

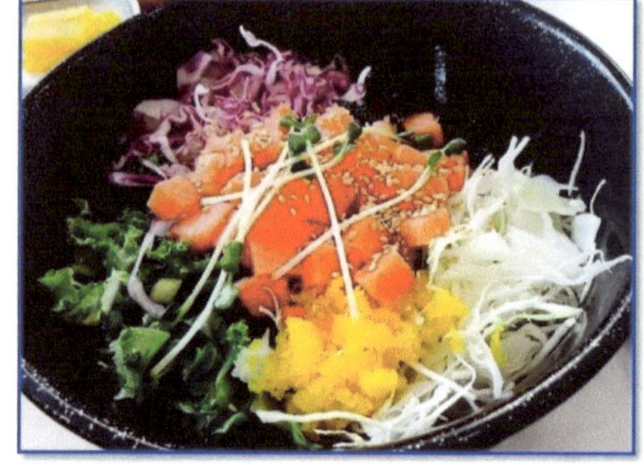

Energy Dense Foods

Energy dense foods contain many calories as compared to their number of nutrients. For example, if you were to eat one 219g McDonald's Big Mac, it contains 563 calories, a whopping 28% of your daily recommended caloric intake. Now that is a lot of calories for just one hamburger that will only be one part of one of your daily meals.

It also contains Vitamin C, 1% of your suggested daily intake, folate at 25% of your suggested daily intake and magnesium at 11% of your suggested daily intake. The ratio of energy to nutrients is comparatively low, and one can imagine that this isn't the healthiest choice.

Nutrient Dense Foods

Nutrient dense foods contain many nutrients compared to the number of calories. For example, if you were to eat a 100g portion of spinach, it contains 188% of your suggested daily Vitamin A intake, 604% of your suggested daily Vitamin K and 49% of your suggested daily folate intake along with other key nutrients. The total number of calories is 23, 1% of your daily recommended caloric intake.

8 Key Benefits Of Whole Food

There are several key benefits that can be derived from eating clean. Here are eight of the more common ones:

1. Improve Your Mood

The Mayo Clinic points out that beyond just affecting weight, eating highly processed foods or those with trans fats can have negative effects on your energy, mood, and the functionality 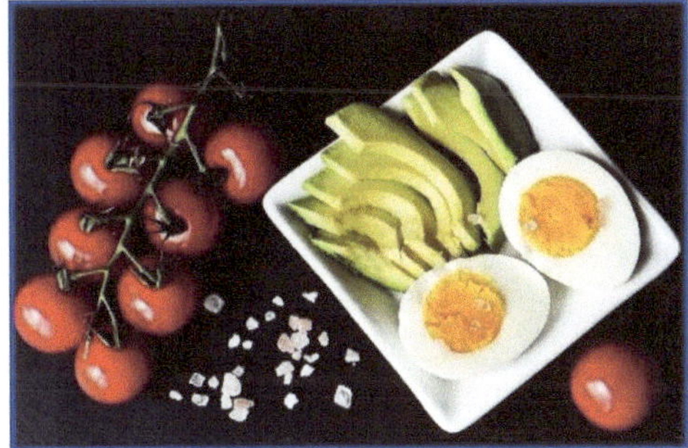 of your brain. Eating a diet primarily composed of these foods can cause you to lose energy and become stressed, irritable, or angry.

Cutting these foods out and replacing them with whole foods can help to provide you with more energy and improve mood.

2. Lower Risk Of Heart Disease

Processed food is typically loaded with salt, bad fats and calories. By consuming more vegetables, whole grains and fruit, you can introduce more fiber in your diet, which researchers have found to greatly reduce your risk of heart disease.

3. Lower Risk Of Developing Diabetes

The World Health Organization reports that a diet rich in grains, fruit, and vegetables can help lower your risk of developing Type 2 diabetes, which is at epidemic levels and primarily caused by poor diet and obesity.

4. Easier To Eat A Balanced Diet

Eating a diet rich in whole food makes it easy to eat well-balanced diet, which promotes good health and vitality.

5. Healthy Weight Management

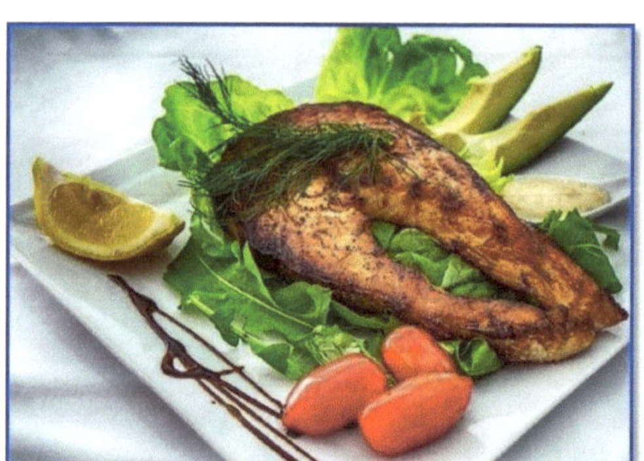

Eating a diet rich in whole food eliminates processed and junk food that is loaded with added fat, sugar and calories.

Eating clean with whole food allows you to enjoy lots of nutrient dense foods versus energy dense foods (high calorie) and therefore manage your weight, lose weight and eat better on the whole.

6. Improve Skin Health

WebMD says that highly-processed foods and foods high in grease, fats, or sugars can cause your complexion to worsen and can actually cause you to break out more frequently.

Introducing more whole foods provides you with key nutrients for all-natural skin health.

7. Increase Your Energy

Whole foods have all the nutrients you need to thrive and have loads of physical and mental energy throughout your busy days.

8. Lengthen Your Life

The Centers For Disease Control advises that highly-processed foods aren't good for you and can, little by little, harm your health, cause obesity and various diet related chronic diseases.

Experts agree that introducing more whole foods into your diet can help to lengthen and improve your life by improving your nutritional profile and therefore greatly improving your health.

Eat Clean To Effectively Lose Weight

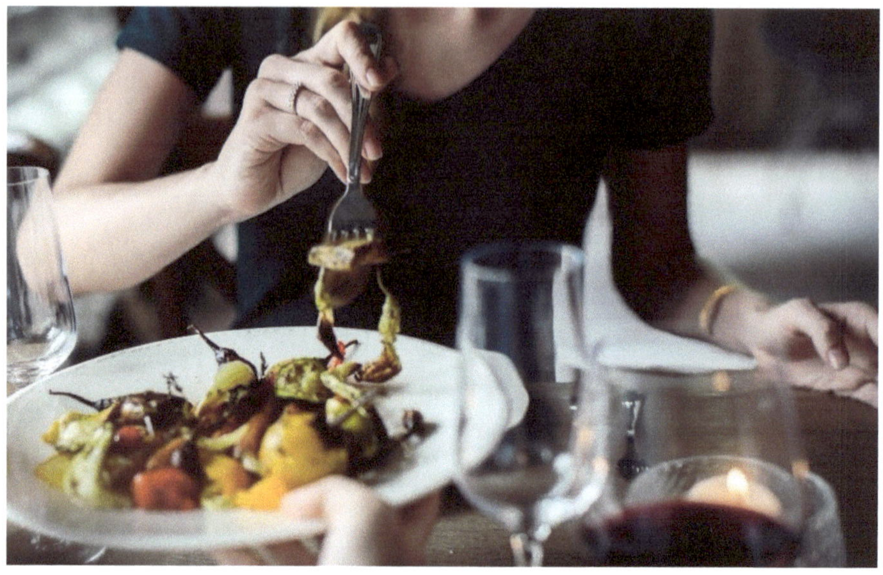

When you switch to a clean eating approach, you will experience numerous health and wellness benefits that will make losing weight easier.

Because you are eliminating some of the significant sources of weight gain from your diet, as well as improving your digestion, your weight loss journey will not only be more accessible but also healthier. Here's why.

You are eliminating a TON of sugar

Added sugar is everywhere these days. From your salad dressing to your cereal, it is pretty difficult sometimes to find a packaged or processed food that doesn't contain added sugars.

But focusing on whole foods, cooking your meals yourself, and eliminating processed products, you will be cutting lots of sugar from your diet.

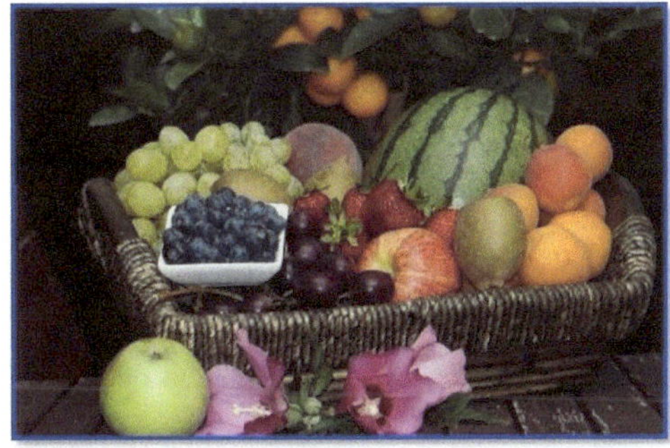

Not only will this reduce the calories you are consuming every day, but you will also be lowering your blood glucose levels as well as your blood pressure.

Sugar is a source of inflammation and, combined with these other issues, can raise your risk of heart disease significantly. So, eliminating sugar, especially added sugars from processed foods, will reap many benefits.

No more refined grains means more fiber.

When you opt for whole grains instead of refined products, you will enjoy the benefits of more fiber in your diet. When you consume more dietary fiber, you are more likely to eat less, stay fuller longer, and have better digestion.

Whole grains also contain other heart-healthy nutrients, like iron and B vitamins, which can improve your health, as well. Eliminating the empty calories of refined grains leaves more room in your diet for tastier, heartier grains that allow you to eat more and weigh less.

Eating less salt means you won't be as likely to overeat.

Like sugar, salt can play tricks on our brain, telling us to eat more, even when we are full. Those who eat a diet high in

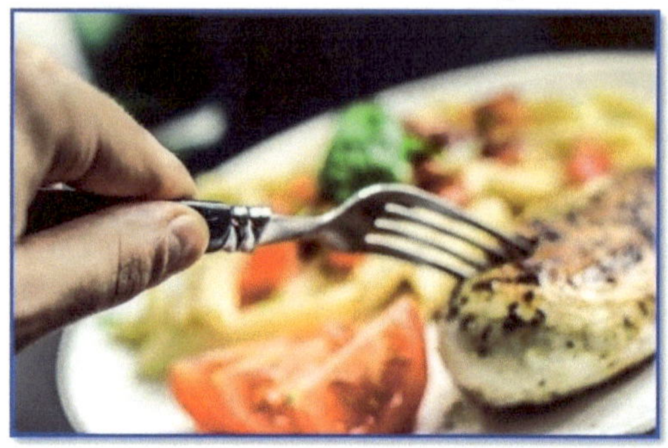

sodium are more likely to overeat, which can lead to weight gain.

When you eliminate processed foods from your diet, you are removing vast amounts of sodium, as nearly every packaged and processed food contains added sodium.

When you prepare your own foods, you control the amount of salt in your diet, and when you use less salt, you are more likely not to over-indulge.

If these reasons are not enough to convince you that eating clean can help you lose weight, consider that whole foods have fewer calories than processed ones, which means you can eat more of them without gaining weight. Keep reading to learn more about how clean eating allows you to eat more and actually weigh less.

Eating Clean Lets You Can Eat More And Weigh Less

When your diet is filled with processed foods, you are often eliminating the food compounds that fill you up and keep you feeling fuller longer.

Processing food adds calories without adding helpful, long-lasting energy.

When you switch to clean eating, you are eating food that fills you up instead of foods that leave you hungry quickly or just make you crave more food. Clean eating can help you shed excess pounds, but it is also healthier for your heart and your digestive system.

To understand how eating more food can help you lose weight, you need to understand calorie density. Some foods contain lots of calories but don't provide you with sustained energy, which means you'll want to eat again soon after consuming them.

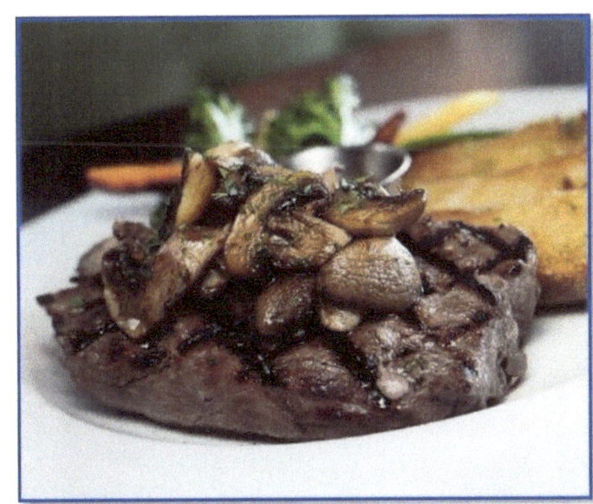

These foods have high calorie density because the serving size is small compared to the number of calories you get. In contrast, foods that are high in fiber and water content offer you lots of energy without a lot of calories.

Each food has a certain number of calories. When you eat high-calorie foods with little water or fiber, as is common in highly-processed foods, you will not get filled up as quickly, which means you will eat more. When you eat low-calorie foods high in fiber or water, as is common in an eating clean approach, you will get fuller faster and stay full longer, which means you will end up eating less.

While 100 calories of apple juice and 100 calories of raw apple have the same amount of energy, you get to eat a lot more apples to get to 100 calories, and you will feel fuller longer after eating that apple than drinking the juice.

In addition to eating more fiber, when you eat cleanly, you will consume less fat. Fat has lots of calories, yet it does not fill you up. A clean eating lifestyle means you are eating healthy fats that are necessary for heart health, but you won't over-indulge in unhealthy fats that get stored in your body and interfere with your weight loss. Eating clean means, you eliminate all the sources of unhealthy fats found in processed foods.

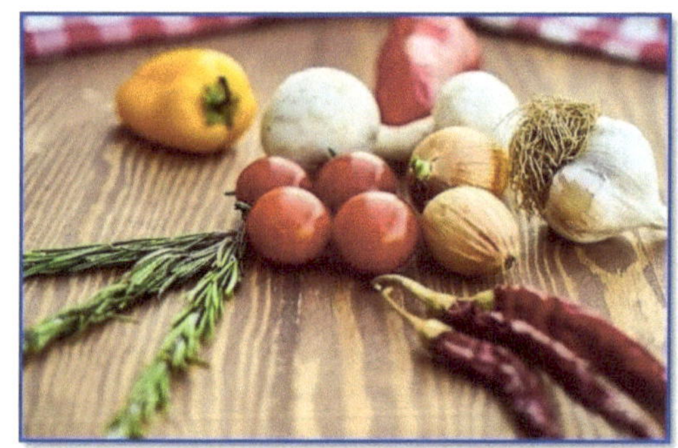

When you eat cleanly, you can consume all the fruit and vegetables you like, as long as they are minimally prepared.

In addition, clean eating includes whole grains and lean proteins that will also ensure you are getting all the minerals and vitamins you need.

These essential nutrients are often removed when food is highly processed. Like vegetables and fruits, whole grains take longer for your body to break down into energy. That means they stay with you longer, giving you a steadier release of energy from glucose.

When foods are highly processed, they are often missing the essential nutrients we all need to be healthy. Fiber is the first component to go, often, when food is processed, and most adults do not get the fiber they need for their digestive or heart health.

Whole foods are going to give you more energy and nutrients than processed foods, which will keep you feeling full and help your body have everything it needs for healthy functions.

Weight Loss And Health Benefits Of Clean Eating

Not only can clean eating help you lose weight, it can promote a healthier heart, lower your risk of cancer, reduce your blood sugar and blood pressure, and support your immune system.

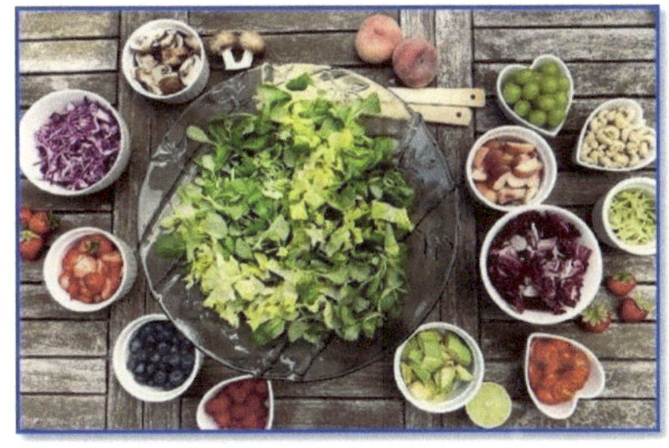

When you switch from highly-processed foods to cleaner options, you are providing your body with all it needs for healthy maintenance without all the added calories and fat of the SAD diet.

Research tells us that a diet rich in high-fiber foods like whole grains, vegetables, nuts, seeds, and legumes, balanced with healthy fats and lean proteins, is the safest, more effective way to lose weight. This diet also supports better health by lowering your risk of heart disease, cancer, type 2 diabetes, and other chronic illnesses.

When you replace unhealthy, highly-processed foods with whole, real foods that have been minimally processed, your body will begin to burn calories and fat more efficiently, your hormones will become balanced to increase your metabolism, and you can more successfully lose the excess weight you have been carrying around.

Diets high in processed foods that contain added sugars and refined carbohydrates create high levels of insulin in your bloodstream. When you eat a primarily SAD diet, your body does not have to work hard to convert food into glucose and then release it into your bloodstream.

This causes your glucose levels to rise, which signals your pancreas to release insulin. Soon, you are in a vicious cycle of insulin production, high blood sugar levels, and insulin resistance in your cells. All this can lead to Type 2 diabetes, and when your diet contains excess sugar and refined carbohydrates, your risk is significantly higher for developing this disease. This also makes it even harder to lose weight.

When you choose healthier, high-fiber carbohydrates, and balance these with other, whole foods, lean proteins, and healthy fats, you can maintain steadier levels of blood sugar and insulin, which promotes better weight loss and long-term health.

Remember that eating clean is all about moderation and variety. For example, while fruit and honey are both clean foods, if you only eat these, you will not lose weight or be healthy. You must balance these with other, less-sugary clean foods in order to maintain healthy blood glucose levels and lose weight.

As with all healthy eating plans, portion size, variety, and moderation will be key to making clean eating work for you and your weight loss goals, but it is the most effective way to lose weight and maintain a healthy weight over time.

Use These 6 Tips To Eat Clean and Maintain Weight Loss For Life

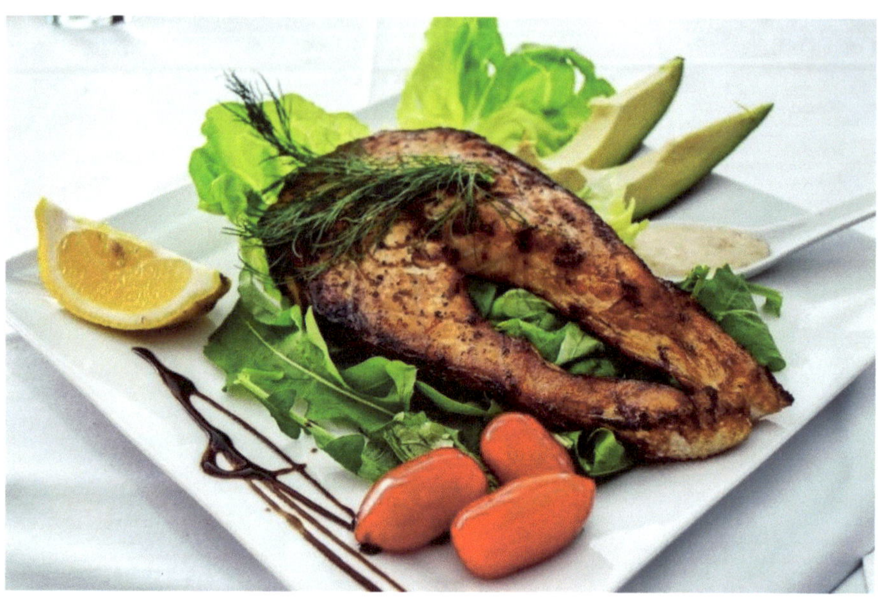

When switching to a clean eating approach and can be difficult to know where to start or how to maintain this lifestyle over time. Here, we offer a collection of tips and hints to help you get started, deal with some of the changes you are likely to encounter when you make a dramatic change such as this, and how to stay successful over time.

Eat More Often

A clean eating approach balances healthy fats, complex carbohydrates, and high-quality proteins.

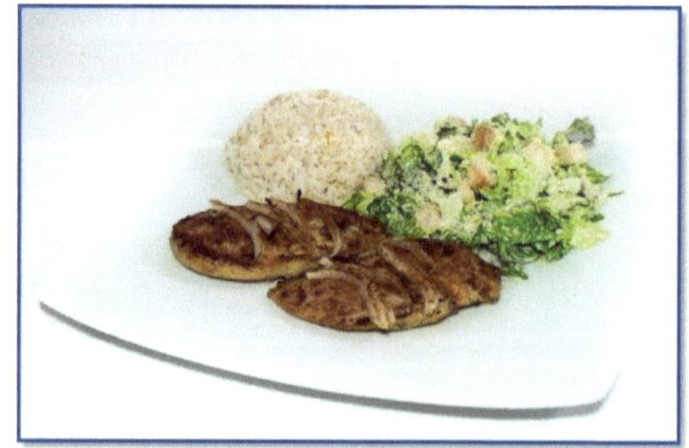

When you eat smaller, more frequent balanced meals and snacks, you provide your body with a more consistent fuel source, which leads to less energy lag.

By only eating three larger meals per day, you set yourself up for dips in your blood sugar, which can have you reaching for sugary snacks and other unhealthy choices. Instead, try to eat at least five times per day in smaller amounts.

Stay Hydrated

When you increase your fiber intake, it is vital that you also drink more water. Drinking at least two liters of water a day will keep your system functioning correctly as well as promote healthy digestion.

Wherever you go, keep a water bottle with you and drink a glass of water with each meal or snack, as well. The health benefits of drinking plenty of water are immeasurable, so don't skimp on this vital part of your healthy, clean eating plan.

Always Have a Plan

One of the biggest shifts you will need to make when you switch to a clean eating lifestyle is how much you should plan for food. In addition to planning and prepping for meals at home, you also need to have a plan for when you are away from your refrigerator.

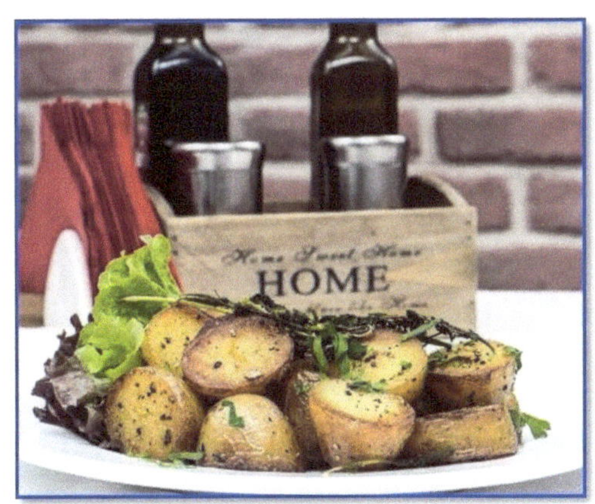

Clean eating is difficult to do when you rely on quick stops at convince stores or lots of lunches on the go. Each week, plan for each meal and snack based on your schedule.

Prepare as much as you can in advance on a day when you are less busy. Each night, pack whatever you need to take with you the next day when you are away from home. Planning for success means you are more likely to stay on track and have access to the clean foods you need.

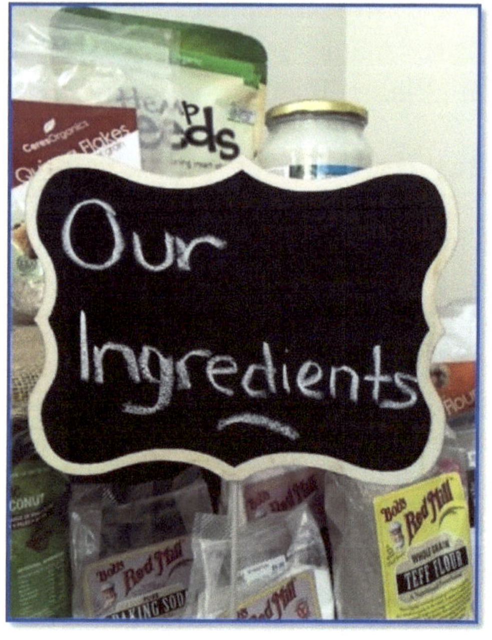

Start Reading Labels

Clean foods are as close to their natural state as possible and shouldn't contain any additives.

If you are purchasing minimally processed foods at the store, always read the labels. Look for ingredients that indicate added sugars or fats or processed foods of any kind.

Say no to foods that contain high fructose corn syrup, colors, dyes, artificial sweeteners, hydrogenated oils, trans fats of any kind, or ingredients with names you cannot pronounce. When possible, go for organic foods and free-range animal products, which will have less exposure to pesticides, herbicides, hormones, or antibiotics, as well.

Watch How You Interact With Other Eaters

Eating clean may be your passion, but not everyone will feel the same. When eating out with other diners, staying on track does not have to be difficult nor does it have to be the focus on the entire meal.

Most restaurants have choices that are clean-eating-friendly or will allow for modifications that allow you to stay on track.

Knowing the menu ahead of time can also be helpful, so you will have a plan in place before you get there. But don't let your newfound healthy focus make others feel bad when dining together. Everyone makes their own choices, so honor that among your fellow diners.

You Won't Be Perfect, And That's Okay

While you can do your absolute best to eat cleanly all the time, there will be times when it can be downright impossible, or you decide it's not the choice you want to make for that meal or snack. Indulging every once in a while, is okay. When you are eating cleanly nearly all the time, the occasional indulgence will not ruin your health.

Often, people find that treats they used to love don't have the same effect after eating cleanly, though, as your tastes change when you get rid of highly-processed foods, so don't be surprised if that piece of cake doesn't taste so good after a while.

Food You Can You Eat On A Clean Diet

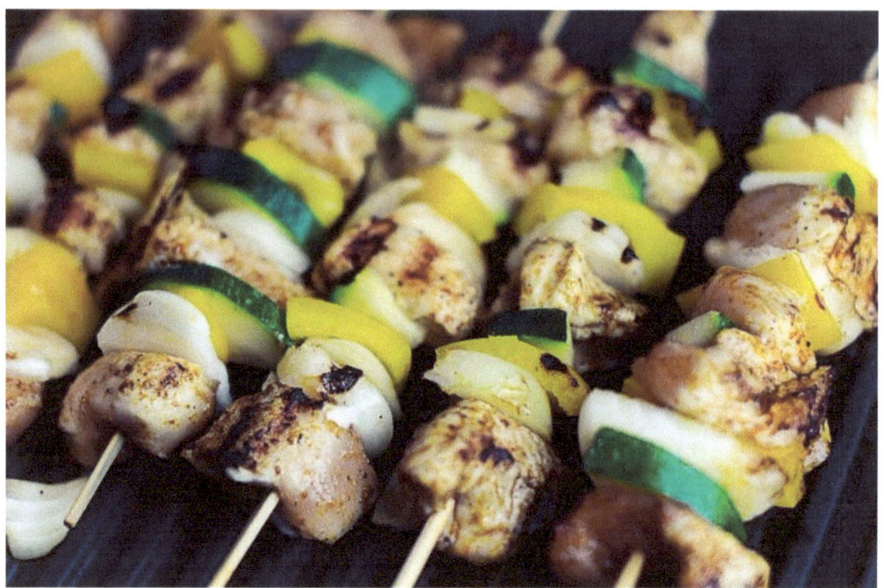

Knowing which foods are acceptable on a clean eating plan is important, as is how those foods should be prepared. Below, we give you the rundown on the best foods to select for your clean eating lifestyle, including some minimally processed options that are acceptable in moderation.

Keeping your pantry, refrigerator, and freezer well stocked with these clean-eating staples will ensure you are able to stick with your plan and prepare meals and snacks that allow you to stay on track with your clean eating lifestyle.

Vegetables

The majority of your clean eating diet should be comprised of fresh vegetables. Vegetables are not only low in calories, but they contain high amounts of fiber and essential vitamins and minerals.

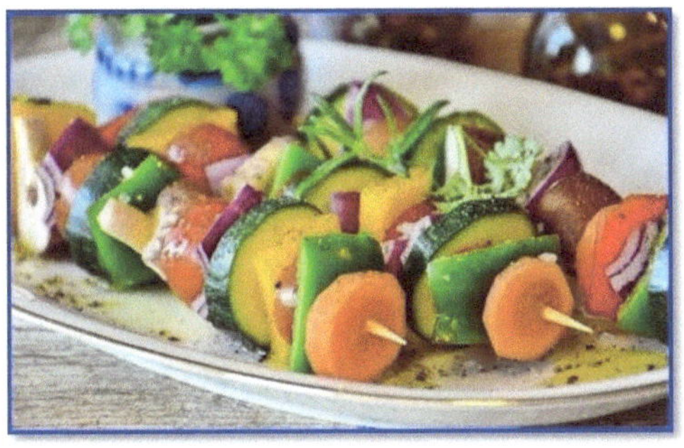

Fresh vegetables are always the best choice, but canned and frozen vegetables are good options, too, as long as they have no added salt and come without sauces or other ingredients.

Some vegetables can be high in calories, like starch potatoes and some winter root vegetables. While you do not necessarily need to limit these in your diet, just be aware that they are higher in calories and have more sugar carbs.

Fruit

Fresh fruit is a clean whole food option for your diet. Fresh fruits are the best choice to make in this category, eaten raw to enjoy their natural goodness. Dried fruits and canned fruits often contain very high levels of sugar, so be sure to read labels and eat these sparingly. These

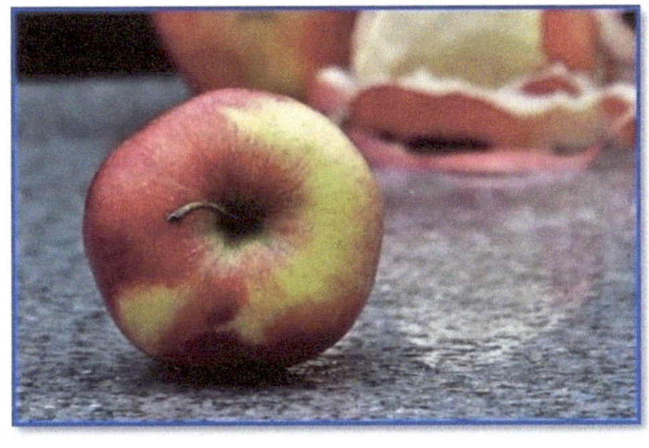

will not fill you up and satisfy your hunger the way fresh fruit will.

Choose fresh whenever possible or choose canned packed water. Frozen without any added ingredients is fine. Dried fruits are best when they are homemade, so you can control your ingredients.

While fruit juice can be used as a serving of fruit, juicing your own is best. Juice does not contain the beneficial fiber of whole fruit, and because you are likely to drink more than just a single serving, you are getting a lot of sugar without a lot of other nutritional benefits. Drink juice only occasionally and eat more whole fruit.

Whole Grains

- 100% whole wheat flour (must be whole wheat not just wheat)

- 100% whole wheat or whole-grain bread, tortillas, hot dog and hamburger buns, etc.

- Ezekiel bread

- 100% whole wheat pasta

- Bob's Red Mill™ offers very clean flour varieties, including almond flour, coconut flour, soy flour and many others

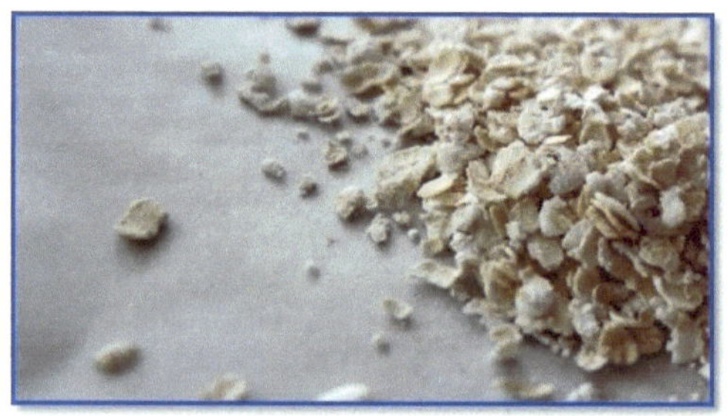

- Amaranth

- Barley

- Brown rice

- Wild rice

- Buckwheat

- Bulgur

- Quinoa

- Rye

- Spelt

- Steel cut oats (no added sugar)

- 100% whole grain cereals, like Kashi™ 7 Whole Grain Flakes, Grape Nuts and others (check ingredients)

Switching from refined grains to whole-grain versions gives you additional dietary fiber, protein, and other nutritional benefits. Grains such as quinoa, barley, brown rice, millet, steel cut oats, and faro are unprocessed. They also contain only one ingredient, making them whole foods.

Popcorn is a whole-grain snack, too. Purchase kernels and cook in an air fryer or on the stove.

If you are opting for a more processed product, like pasta, bread, or flour-based products, read ingredients carefully. Whole-wheat flour should be the first ingredient, and there should not be any added sugar or other processed ingredients on the list. Sprouted-grain breads are an even better choice, as long as they adhere to these same guidelines.

Dairy

- Eggs (pasture raised/grass fed or organic)

- Organic milk or milk from grass fed cows

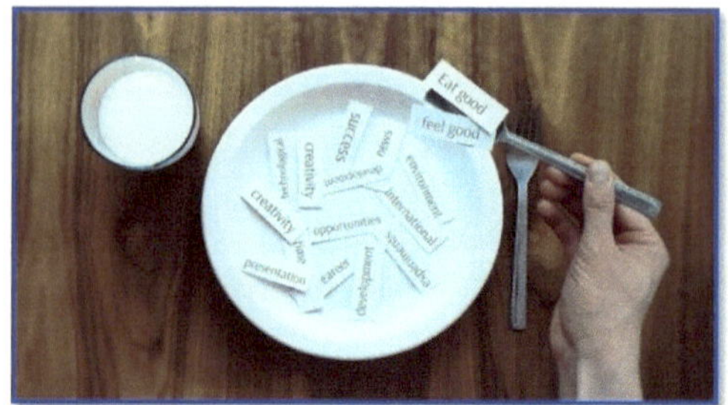

- Nut milks (without added sugar)

- Soy milks (without added sugar)

- Organic Greek yogurt

- Organic soy yogurt

- Cottage cheese

- Sour cream

- Block cheeses (shredded adds a chemical to keep the cheese separated)

Like other food categories, always opt for the fewest ingredients with no added sugars. Plain yogurt and natural or raw cheeses are preferred to sweetened or flavored varieties. If you enjoy alternatives to dairy milk, read the labels and select those with no added sugar and minimal additional ingredients.

Lean Protein

Beef and Chicken

- Fresh red meat (steaks, hamburger, ribs and roasts)

- Fresh pork (steaks and roasts)

- Fresh chicken

- Bison or venison

- Fresh turkey

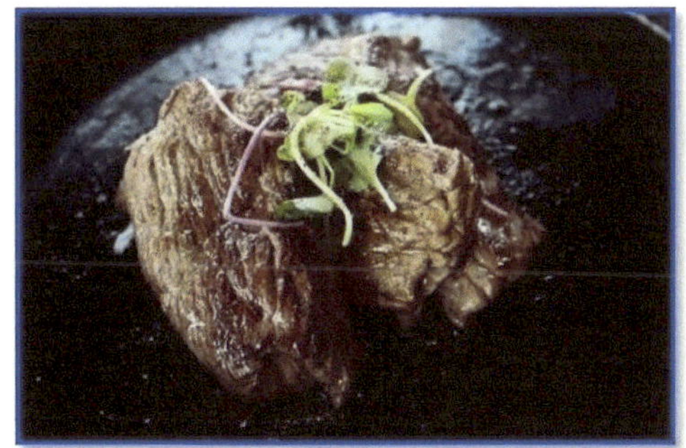

Fish and Seafood

All fresh fish and seafood, preferably wild caught versus farm raised

Plant Based

Choosing plant-based sources of protein more often allows you to naturally lower caloric intake in your diet, these include:

- Beans

- Seeds

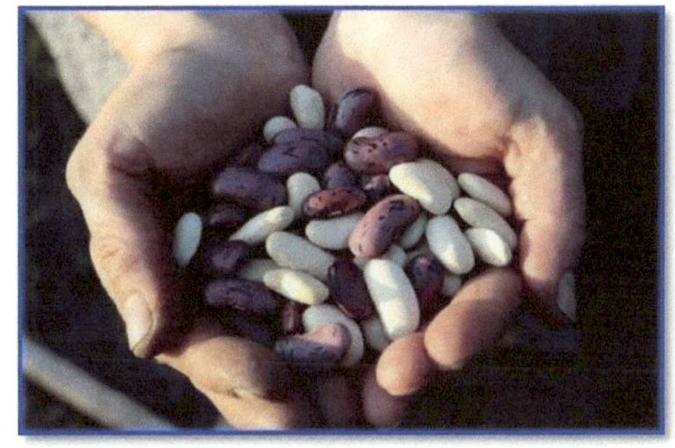

- Nuts

- Nut butters

- Soy products and soy milk

Be sure to buy whole foods with no added salt. Buying dried beans is not only less expensive but also means you are getting the benefit of a whole food with no additional ingredients.

When selecting meat products, opt for leaner cuts and types of animals for single-ingredient meats. Avoid cured or processed meats of all kinds.

Fish and seafood are excellent choices that provide healthy fats, as well. Eggs are not only an excellent source of protein but also essential nutrients.

In all cases, look for grass-fed animal sources raised using organic practices. Grass fed, pasture raised, or organic meat is always best as it is devoid of antibiotics and growth hormones fed to traditionally-farmed animals.

Fats

- Grass fed butter

- Avocados

- Walnuts

- Olive oil

- Nut oils

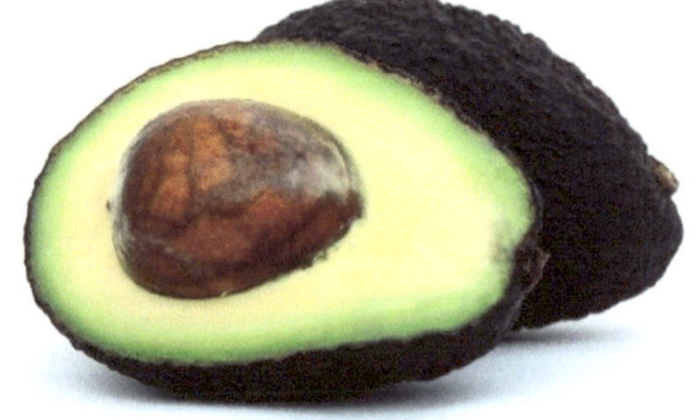

- Grapeseed oil

For desserts choose whole whipping cream versus manufactured whipped topping products

Packaged and Snack Foods

The best choices will have the "Non-GMO Project Verified" seal. Look at labels to check ingredients. Stores like Trader Joe's™ and Whole Foods™ are good places to find many whole food/clean eating packaged items.

- Sun-dried tomatoes

- KIND™ Snacks

- RX™ Bars

- LARA™ Bars - these snack bars list their very simple whole ingredients right on front of the package in big bold print

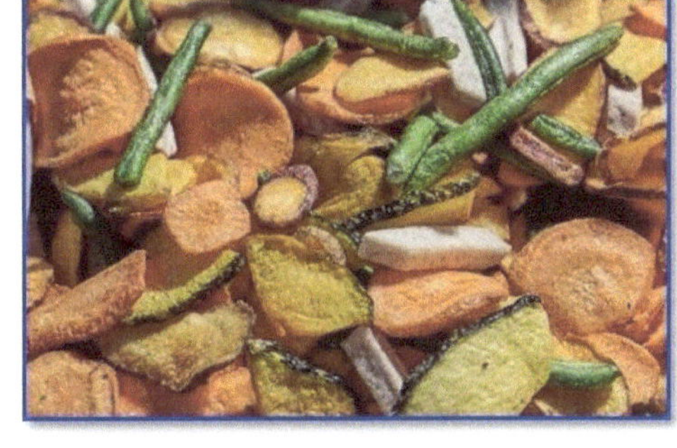

- Vegetable chips – a new trend in healthy snacking, you can find green bean, kale, beet and carrot chips, the best ones will have two ingredients, the vegetable and oil. You can also make your own.

- 100% Pure Nut Butters - peanut, almond and others are available in brands where the ingredients list is the nut and nothing else

- Air popped popcorn (check ingredients for anything else added)

- Raisins, prunes and all dried fruit (as long as nothing else is added, especially sugar, dried fruit is also very high in fruit sugars and should be eaten in moderation, fresh is better)

- All nuts (plain, raw and unflavored)

- All seeds (plain, raw and unflavored)

- 60% +cacao dark chocolate

- Unsweetened cocoa powder

Beverages

- Water

- Milk and nut milks

- Naturally sweetened coffee & tea

- Freshly squeezed juices (fruit and vegetable)

- Seltzers/Club Soda (without added sugar)

- 100% pure coconut milk (high in calories, use in moderation)

- Wine (in moderation)

- Beer (in moderation)

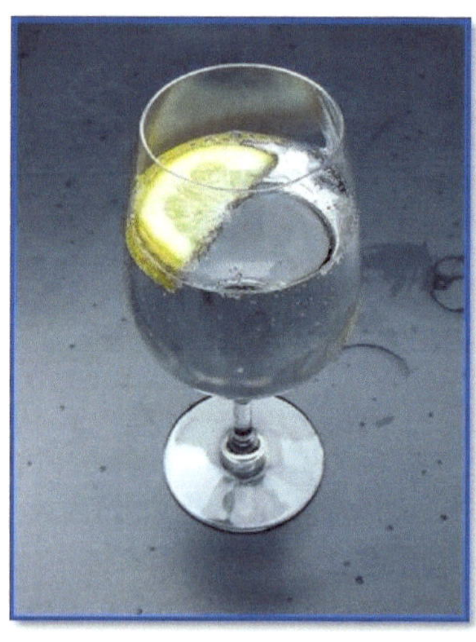

8 Tips To Get Started With Clean Eating

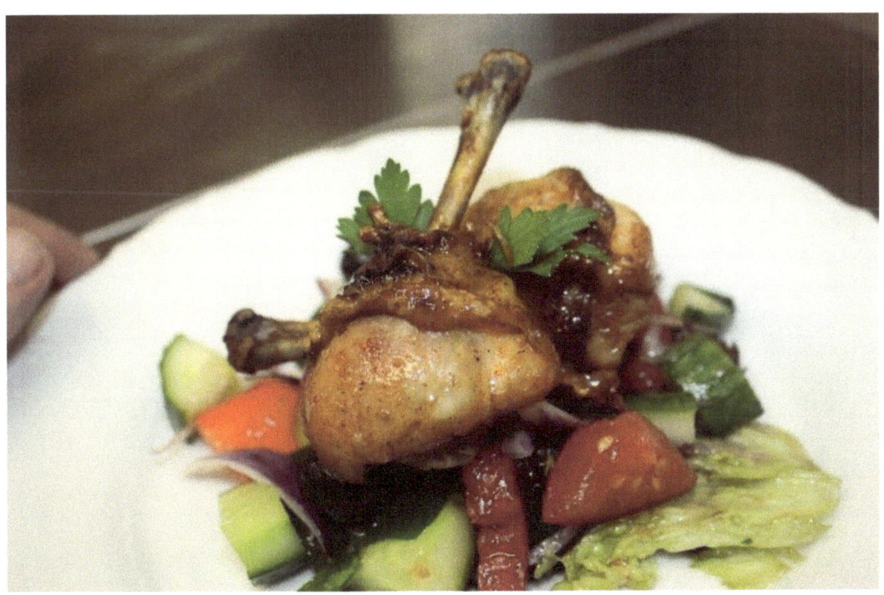

Do you need more help getting started with the clean eating approach? Below are additional strategies that can help you be successful with a clean eating lifestyle.

Eat Whole Food

Keep food preparation simple and use few ingredients per dish (less is more).

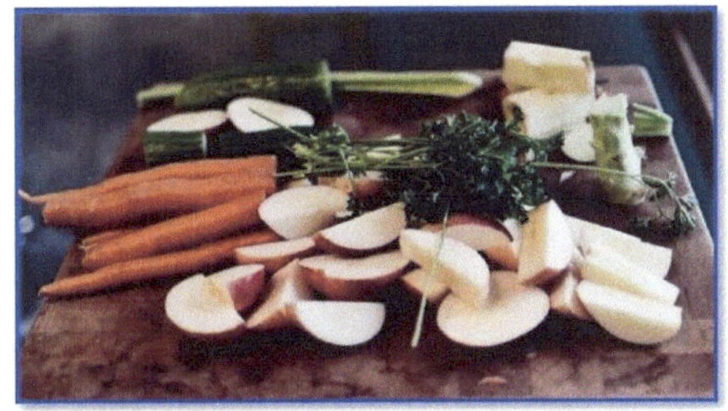

When eating out, pick simple choices, like a salad, plain meats etc.

Shop at your local farmers market, for seasonal, fresh and delicious produce.

Don't go into the aisles of the grocery store – the simple, healthy foods are at the perimeter.

Avoid

- Processed salamis, meats and sausages, fish sticks, chicken fingers

- Juices, fruit concentrates, jams with sugars and additives and canned fruits in syrup

- Salted and roasted nuts, potato chips and similar snacks

- Sweets, candies, chocolate and gum

- Bought sauces and marinades etc.

- All store-bought energy dense foods are processed!

Gradual Steps

When you are ready to begin with a clean eating approach to your food, start small and take gradual steps. Throwing all your food away at once and changing all aspects of your diet at once is a recipe for failure. Instead, identify a few areas of your diet to improve, and make those first steps.

Focusing on just a few things each day you can change means your transformation will be gradual and also something you can live with. Your goal is to create a lasting lifestyle change, which takes time and buy-in from you.

Once you start to change the way you eat, your tastes will adjust, too, and you'll notice you are craving your old foods less and less.

Making healthy, clean swaps for some of your favorite foods

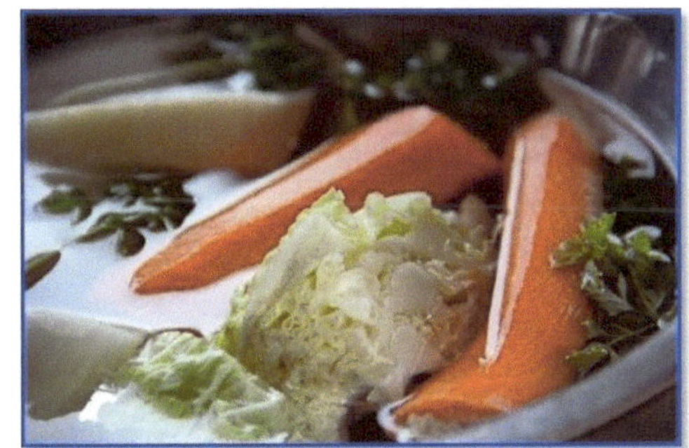

is easy, and just making a few at a time means you won't feel deprived or wind up thinking constantly about your food. Each one of the changes is positive and will add up to a clean lifestyle before you know it.

Cook For Yourself

When you cook all your own food, you know exactly what is going into it.

You control the sugar, salt, and fat in your meals and snacks, and you'll know precisely how processed and refined your food really is. When cooking isn't possible, go for the dish that contains the most whole-food items and ask for no additional butter or oil to be used in preparing your food. Better yet, opt for raw options.

Choose Whole Foods Over Processed Versions

This may seem like a no-brainer, but it bears repeating. When you buy foods that come in a box or have a package, you aren't just getting food, in most cases. You are also likely getting chemicals or additives.

Stick to whole foods whenever possible, and you will avoid eating the fats, sugars, salt, and preservatives that are making modern society sick and fat.

Clear Your Kitchen of Processed Foods

Go through your pantry, refrigerator, and freezer and identify anything that is highly-processed. If there are foods you just can't live without, seek out less-processed versions or find ways to make them yourself using whole ingredients.

Look carefully at everything in your kitchen that has a box, wrapper, or other packaging. If it isn't a whole food or contains these unhealthy, added ingredients, consider donating it and getting it out of your house over time.

Focus Each Meal On Balance

When you include healthy fat, protein, and carbohydrates at every meal, along with lots of vegetables, you will be giving your body the complete nutrition it needs to thrive. Finding foods that include more than one of the macro-nutrients is even better.

For example, quinoa is an excellent whole grain that also has protein, so it makes an excellent choice for eating clean. Your fats should come from a variety of natural sources and include different unsaturated fats as well as some saturated ones.

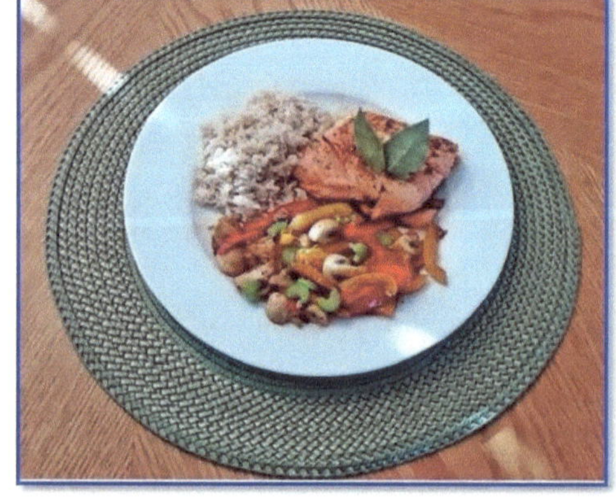

Be sure to get sufficient amounts of omega-3 fatty acids. If you keep this focus in mind every time you eat, you'll feel less hungry and have a more rounded diet with better variety.

Watch What You Drink

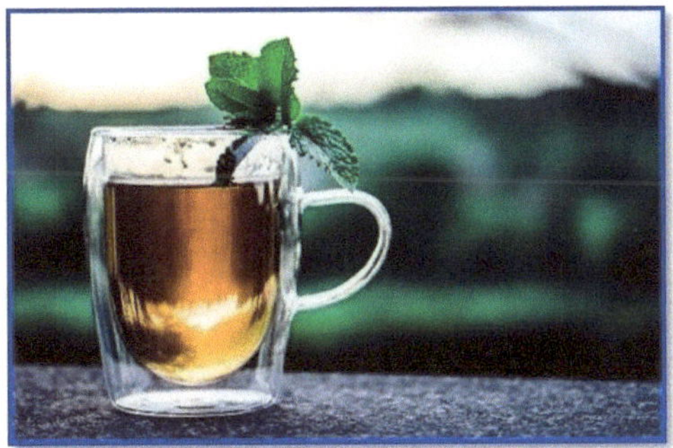

Just as being aware of what is in your food is important, so is watching what you drink. Water will always be your best choice when it comes to beverages, and you need plenty of it on a clean-eating meal plan.

Water keeps hunger at bay, aids in digestion, and provides all your organs and muscles the necessary hydration for proper function.

Avoid sweetened beverages of any kind, as well as caffeinated drinks and alcohol. Soda and fruit juice contain high amounts of empty calories from sugar with little or no nutritional benefits. Alcohol turns to glucose in your system, raising your blood sugar levels and providing no nutrients.

If you drink sugary soda every day, start by cutting back on the number you drink. When you are down to one a day, start mixing your soda with sparkling water until you are just drinking water. Or, switch to sparkling water mixed with a bit of fresh fruit. If you love a specific dish that you used to make with lots of convenience foods, find a recipe that uses only whole ingredients and practice making it at home until you are happy with the results.

A Typical Day of Clean Eating

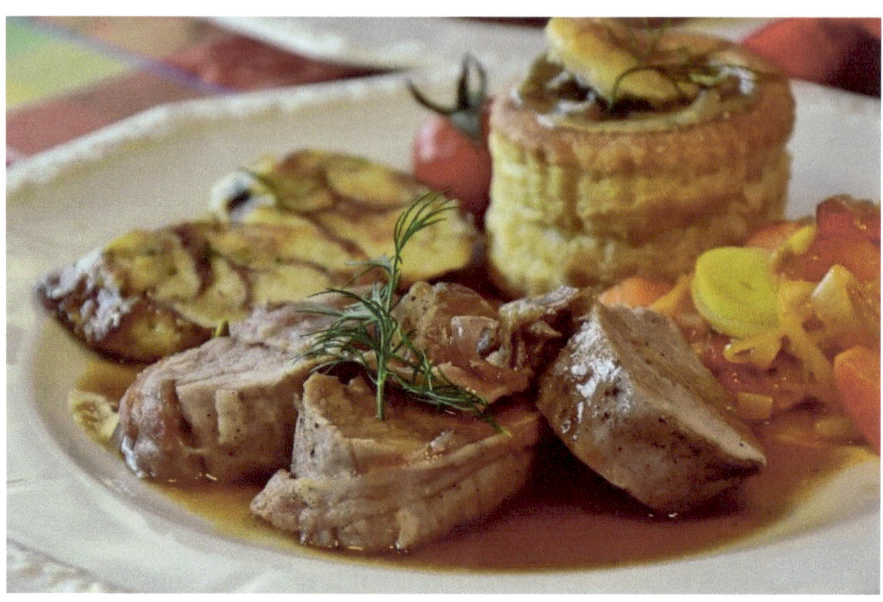

- **Breakfast**- An omelet made from one whole egg, two egg whites, and chopped vegetables including spinach, tomatoes, and onions. Use fresh herbs or salt-free seasoning to taste. Enjoy with one slice of whole-grain toast.

- **Snack**- One-half of a sprouted-grain English muffin topped with one tablespoon natural almond butter and one-half of a banana, sliced.

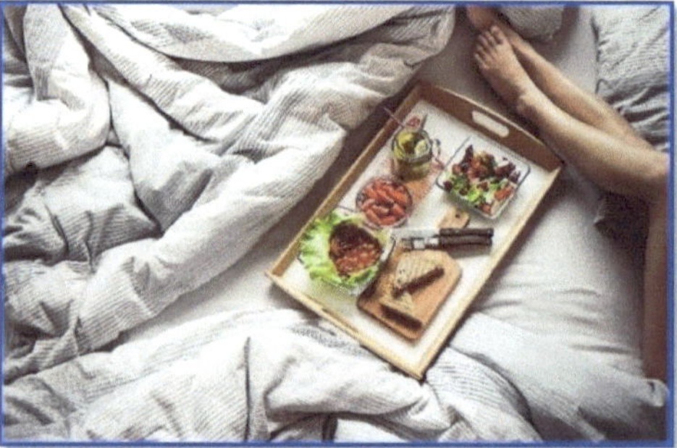

- **Lunch**- Salad greens topped with chickpeas, one-half of a small avocado sliced, and chopped fresh vegetables. Drizzle with homemade vinaigrette and enjoy with one-quarter cup of cottage cheese and one-quarter cup of diced fresh pineapple.

- **Snack**- Two cups of air-popped popcorn

- **Dinner**- Five ounces of grilled salmon with one-half cup wild rice, and roasted Brussels sprouts.

- **Snack**- One orange, sliced and sprinkled with cinnamon

How to Whole Food Shop

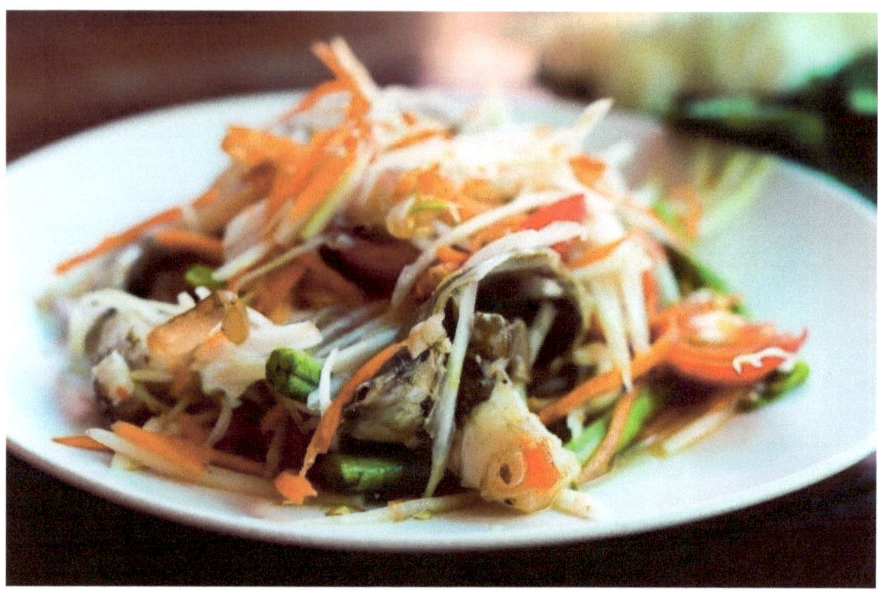

What you SHOULD NOT buy:

- Refined grains

- White flour and foods made with them

- White starches, like pasta, rice or breads

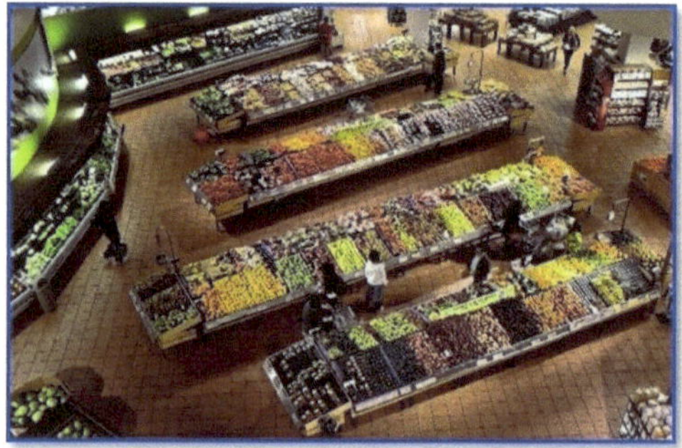

- Refined sugars

- Table sugar

- Sweets, like cakes cookies, ice cream, soda etc.

- Anything that comes in a bag, box, bottle or package that has more than 5 ingredients, preferably less than 4, and none of those should contain trans fats or a lot of sugar

- Anything not from the outer periphery of the supermarket

- Deep fried foods

- Fast food junk

6 Strategies You Can Use To Deal With Junk Food Cravings

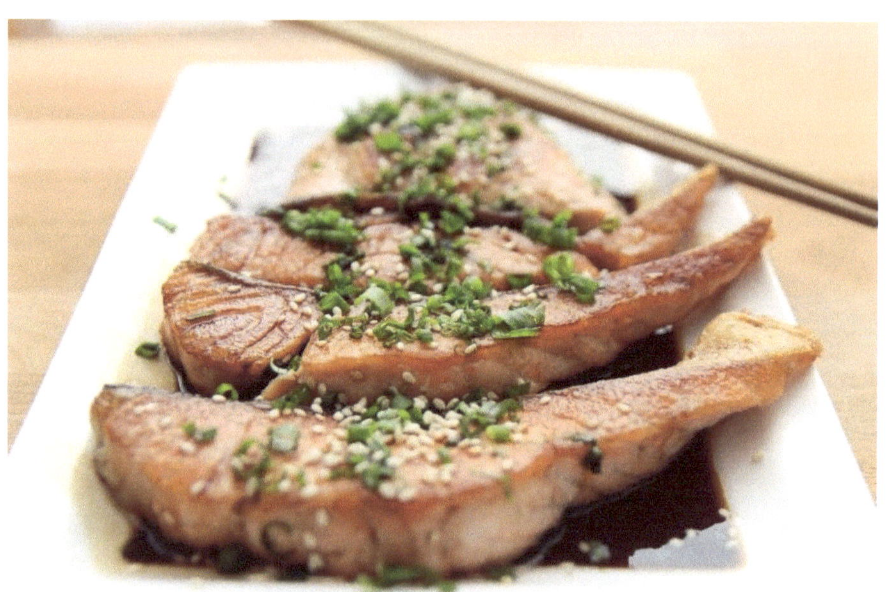

When you switch to a clean eating approach, you may find, especially in the beginning, that you still crave some of your old, highly-processed favorites. Your brain's dependence on sugar and salt can be quite high, especially if your previous diet contained a lot of processed foods. Here are some tips for dealing with those junk food cravings.

Don't Wait Until You Are Starving

This is key, as when you are famished you are much more likely to make bad food choices. Extreme hunger can lead to cravings. If you notice you are starting to feel hungry, it's better to eat a small snack than wait until you are extremely hungry. This will also help you maintain a more consistent blood glucose level, which keeps cravings at bay, too.

Drink More Water

We often confuse hunger for thirst. When you find you are really longing for something to eat, drink a glass of water first. Wait a bit. In many cases, your craving will disappear.

Eat Some Protein

Hunger and cravings can sometimes be a cue that you are not getting the protein you need. Remember to balance every meal and snack, including small amounts of protein at each one. Protein helps you feel fuller and more satisfied, so nibble on a high-protein snack if you are hankering for junk food and include protein with each meal and snack to reduce the urge to snack altogether.

Get Up and Move

If you are craving a snack, try to take your mind off it by taking a walk or doing something different for a bit. Switching your activity will often get your mind off its focus on food.

Have a Plan

Having a plan for what you'll eat is very helpful for dealing with cravings. It means you'll have snacks stocked and ready to go when the craving strikes, making you less likely to reach for a convenience food instead.

Make Sure You Are Sleeping

Fatigue and tiredness are significant contributors to cravings. When you don't sleep well, your hormones can become imbalanced, which can lead to cravings.

Not sleeping also impacts your eating patterns, which can lead to hunger and cravings, as well. Getting sufficient sleep is essential for all body functions, including hunger and digestion.

Final Thoughts

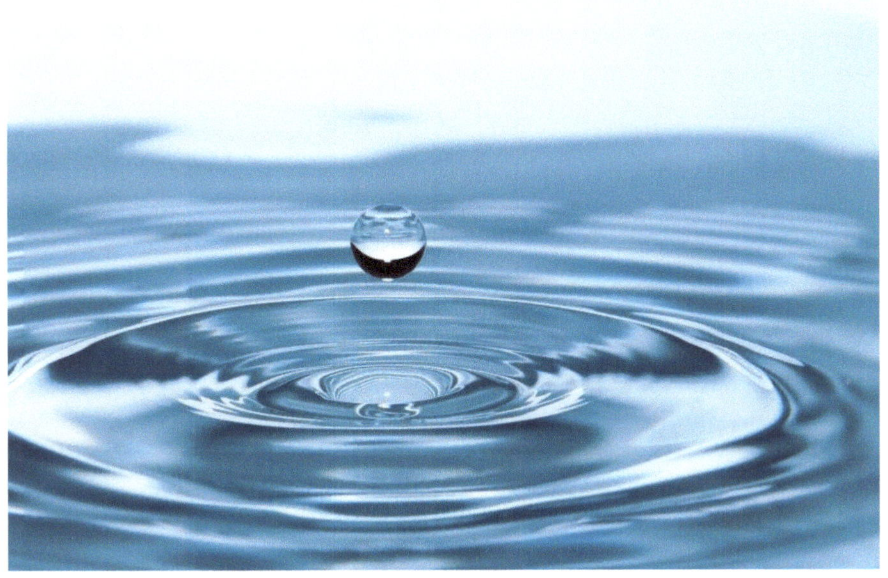

When choosing a clean eating approach to your life, your body will benefit from getting plenty of fiber and essential nutrients through meals and snacks that do not contain added ingredients and that are minimally processed.

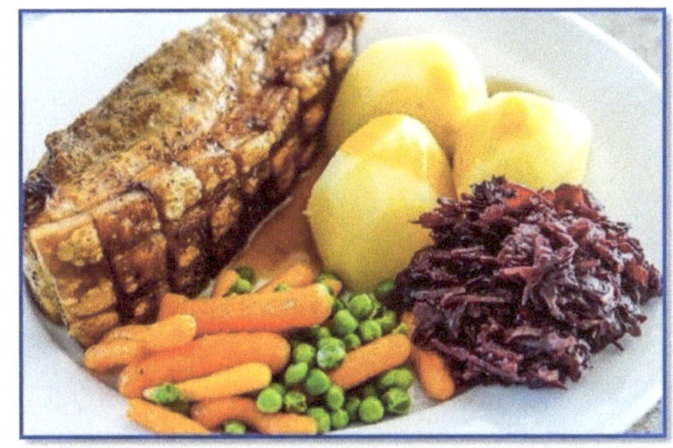

When you eat the majority of your calories from vegetables, fruits, whole grains, healthy fats, and lean proteins that are minimally processed, your body can absorb all the nutrients available, and your weight and overall health will benefit greatly.

For centuries, we ate food in its natural form or with minimal preparation. It is only since we altered our diet to include added sugars, fats, salts, and chemicals that we have seen a dramatic increase in obesity, heart disease, diabetes, and other chronic illnesses. A return to the clean, whole-foods approach to eating and help solve many of these problems.

Other Relevant Books by This Author

If you would like to read more relevant books about this topic, here is a list of the CreateSpace links, titles and descriptions from this author:

https://www.amazon.com/Mindful-Eating-Mindfully-Emotional-Physical/dp/1975988930

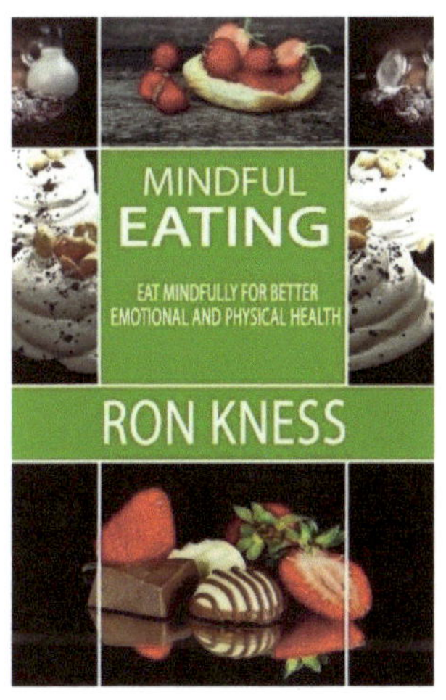

Mindful Eating: Eat Mindfully for Better Emotional and Physical Health

This Guide Could Be Your Key To Better Health!

What type of person are you when it comes to eating? There's two main types of eaters in this world, there's the type who are conscious of every bite they put in their mouth ... and then there's the people who eat without realizing what or how much they are eating. Which type of person are you? If you are the latter type, this book is for you. It's 100% your choice.

But frankly, if you're struggling with your emotional health, physical health, or both, learning how to eat mindfully could help improve it. If all of your efforts to resolve your health problems have not yielded the results you have been looking for, what do you have to lose!

In this guide, we ... - Define Mindful (and Mindless) Eating - Talk About Why Junk and Processed Food Is So Addictive - Discuss the 6 Pillars of Mindful Eating - Gain an

Understanding the 7 Different Types of Hunger - Discover How Much Food You Really Need - Deal with Withdrawal, Cravings and Slip-Ups - Learn How to Live and Move Mindfully to Complement Our Your New Eating Program

And the Mindful Eating Guide is complemented by 5 other free downloads, making it a complete eating program ... - Junk Food Alternatives - Healthy Foods List - Mindful Questions to Ask Yourself Before Eating - Training Your Brain - Mindful Eating Checklist

Get your copy today!

https://www.amazon.com/Science-Slimming-Down-Exercising-Nutrition/dp/1542328012

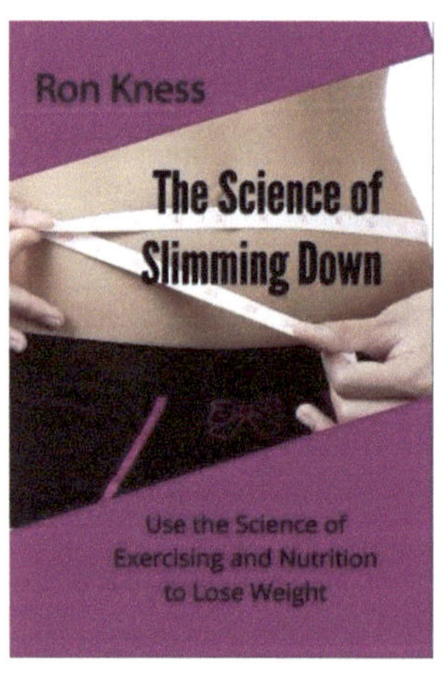

The Science of Slimming Down: Use the Science of Exercising and Nutrition to Lose Weight

Are you carrying a little extra weight around the middle? Maybe you've got more than just a little weight problem – maybe it's a rather large one and you need to get rid of the fat for health reasons. Rest assured that you're not alone!

Obesity in America is at an all-time high. One of out of every three Americans is obese – a number that has doubled in just ten years. This epidemic is growing out of control in other countries as well as fast food franchises open in China, Japan, Germany, and other industrialized nations. When you are overweight, it's a serious issue.

Carrying extra weight can make you more susceptible to heart and joint problems, diabetes, stroke, and various types of cancer. It can also affect your body image as well, thus causing problems with your self-esteem. You deserve to be healthier and take off some of that weight that is making you unhealthy.

But what if you're like me and love food so you hate the idea of having to eat rice cakes and alfalfa sprouts, or starving yourself just to help the weight come off. We have good news for you! You don't have to starve yourself to lose weight! You can still eat in a way that is satisfying, but healthy at the same time.

Many people associate weight loss with being hungry all the time. They're afraid to start a weight loss plan because they want to avoid the frustrations of hunger.

*** The key though, is to not be on a "diet", because once the diet ends, and you go back to your old eating habits, you will regain all the weight you lost (and more). The secret is to change to a new healthy eating lifestyle – one that lasts forever. ***

I show you how in my book - how to eat a healthy nutritious diet that won't leave you hungry coupled with a sensible exercise plan that will result in lasting weight loss. What do you have to lose!

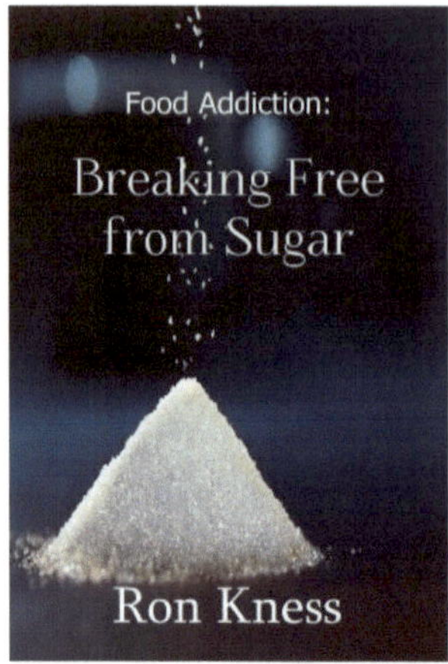

Food Addiction: Breaking Free from Sugar: How and Why You Should Cut Sugar from Your Diet

The thought of eliminating sugar from your diet may seem like torture but actually, it is one of the healthiest things you can do for yourself. Processed sugar acts like a drug to the body adding no nutritional value to your diet - just empty calories.

Most people eat an enormous amount of sugar each day, usually in processed foods such as cereal and soft drinks. Processed sugar is thought to be contributing factor in health issues such as obesity, heart disease, and diabetes. Each teaspoon of sugar contains 4 grams of sugar, which by the way equates to 16 calories.

Most people eat more than 22 grams (5.5 teaspoons) of sugar each day. Too much sugar can cause obesity, heart disease, liver damage, tooth decay and a whole host of other health conditions.

In this book we show you how to recognize hidden sugar, how to break free and detox from the addiction and reduce or eliminate sugar from your diet. Take control and break free from sugar!

About the Author

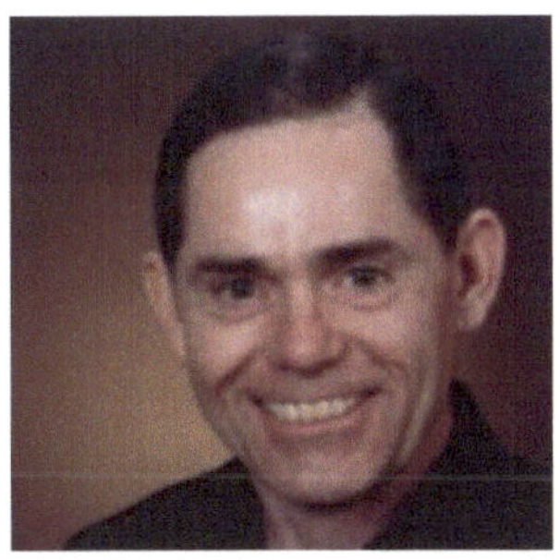

I have published numerous books on Amazon for Kindle, CreateSpace and other publishing platforms.

While most of my books are on health and fitness in general, as I age (now 65) at the time of this writing) my topics of interest are geared toward aging baby boomers and older.

Besides my own writing, I also ghostwrite ebooks, books, reports, articles, blogs and do Kindle conversions for clients on a variety of topics.

Today my wife and I are retired from our careers and live in Gold Canyon, AZ. I now write as a retirement business where you'll find me happily sitting in my office typing away on my laptop as I work on my next book or ghostwriting project . . . that is if we are not traveling on a cruise ship - our new-found mode of travel.